A Complete Lean and Green Cookbook for Beginners

Easy and delicious recipes to build your body, taking advantage of having healthy meals with the best tricks.

Claudia Giordano

Table of Content

Introduction

There are many diets on the market, and there are many cookbooks that relate to them, so it's easy to become confused and mix up what's what. And, when you are researching lifestyle changes that combine diet and exercise, you can become even more confused. So, I am pleased to introduce you to a diet and exercise plan that is so easy to follow, and is totally different to anything you may have seen before. Let's take the confusion right out of the picture; I want to introduce you to Lean and Green. What is it that makes this method of eating different from other diet styles? The frequency of the meals in your plan (up to six per day), and the "fueling" snacks that you will eat in addition to each carefullybalanced meal ensure that you are never hungry, and never lacking in essential fuel to give you energy.

Eating like this is a way to maximize your intake of supernutritious foods, while reaching and maintaining a healthy weight, and this cookbook contains recipes that work perfectly with the tried and tested method that will help you make a difference to your health and without locking you into self-deprivation. Lean and Green meals are high protein and low carbohydrate, which is a very healthy way to eat.

Because most people consider beginning a new diet in order to lose excess weight, it's probably best to start the Lean and Green diet on the start-up plan. You could lose up to twelve pounds (5.4

kg) of excess fat over a twelve-week period. Unlike some other diet plans, this is a way to lose excess weight quickly, without compromising your health or feeling tired because you are not eating enough. On the Lean and Green diet, you eat "fuelings", and one Lean and Green meal, every day. You should also incorporate thirty minutes of moderate exercise, at least four days each week. In this beginning phase, the total food intake (including the fuelings and the meal) should contain no more than 100 grams of carbohydrate each day.

The Basics of Lean and Green Diet

Lean and Green is a diet program that involves a combination of fresh foods, and pre-prepared foods and snacks. Lean and Green also offers additional help from a designated support person. Once you have completed your twelve-week start-up plan, your average Lean and Green meal should then include five to seven ounces of cooked lean protein, plus three servings of non-starchy vegetables, and up to two servings of healthy fats. The plan is to eat up to six meals throughout the day.

If you wish to lose more weight than you lose in the first phase, you can stay on the initial diet plan longer, until you reach your target weight. Once you have reached that weight, you should safely enter the "transition phase." This involves slowly increasing your overall daily food intake to no more than 1,550 calories per day, while adding a wider variety of foods, which will include whole grains, fruits, and low-fat dairy products such as yogurt and cheese. The Lean and Green diet also provides additional tools to aid weight loss and maintenance, which includes tips and inspiration, community forums, weekly support calls, and an app that allows you to set meal reminders to track your food intake and your activity level.

What is Lean and Green Diet?

In short, the Lean and Green diet is designed to help people lose weight and fat by reducing calories and carbs through portioncontrolled meals and snacks. Its basis is reduced carb. programs that combine processed, packaged calorie-counted foods with homemade meals which encourage weight loss. You can choose from several options, which all include products called "fuelings" as well as homemade meals, which follow the Lean and Green carb-fat ratio. The fuelings comprise over sixty items which are low in carbs, but high in protein and probiotic cultures. These friendly bacteria can boost your gut health. These fuelings include snack bars, cookies, shakes, puddings, cereals, soups, and pastas. All super- convenient and nutritious, while designed to help you feel satisfied.

What Do You Eat on Lean and Green Diet?

It's the first question that people always ask about a new diet: "What will I be eating?" Because food is important to us all. It is not only essential to our life, it is pleasurable and sociable. Most of us are used to eating a range of foods from all the essential groups, but we all have to confess that we have our favorites, and our pet hates! So, firstly, let me reassure you, by telling you what you won't be eating: there is nothing in the Lean and Green diet that is "weird", unusual or just boring and unappetizing! You will be eating a huge selection of natural, nourishing foods; foods that you are already used to preparing and eating. The weight-loss secret lies in the planning, support, and the execution of the program that you will be choosing to suit your needs and preferences.

The Lean and Green diet plan includes two weight loss programs, in addition to a carefully balanced weight maintenance plan. So, to answer this question: what you eat, how frequently you eat it, and how much of it you will be eating, depends totally on which of the plans that you are on, and at which stage of the plan you are on at any given time.

A lot of diets that are on the market are successful only because they radically limit the types of food that you are allowed to eat, and how you are able to cook or combine them. Lean and Green doesn't do this, because we think that this way to eat can become rather boring eventually. So, now you don't have to worry about that, there are no unpleasant surprises in store when you choose to eat Lean and Green! The wide variety, and the numerous styles of food that you will be enjoying will keep you feeling nourished and happy to continue. This specialized cookbook will help you to prepare and include all of the readily available, lowcost, popular foods which should always appear in any healthy diet. What's more, using Lean and Green, you will be eating a lot of familiar, nourishing, scrummy foods at selected intervals throughout the day, which will help you to enrich your body while you are losing excess unhealthy weight.

You will still be able to eat those lovely lean cuts of your favourite meats, like chicken, pork and beef. No limits on the amounts of greens and non-starchy vegetables that you consume either. You can tuck into cabbage, kale, cauliflower, broccoli, asparagus, and zucchini. You not limited to fat-free food either. On this diet you will be eating tasty foods which contain healthy fats. Fats like olive and nut oil for cooking and salad dressing are good.

If you are not vegan, you will be able to eat lots of low-fat dairy foods. Yummy yogurts and tasty cheeses are not off-limits! Fresh eggs, low-fat milk and frozen desserts are OK too. Lots of lovely fresh fruits are OK. Thumbs up to crisp apples, juicy oranges, sweet, grapes, zesty pineapples, and energizing bananas! Finally, to help to keep you feeling satisfied throughout the day, the Lean and Green diet naturally includes those comforting, life-giving, delicious essential whole grains and seeds. It's all well-balanced, convenient, and it tastes good!

What is Fueling?

Fueling is a measured, calorie-controlled way of snacking, and it helps you to maintain your energy levels, as well as feeling full throughout the day. More specifically, regular fuelings ensure that you are correctly nourished for your activity levels, whether you are working at your job, or working out. Correctly consumed fuelings provide you with the assurance that you won't be losing essential muscle mass while you are on the Lean and Green diet, because with carefully prepared fueling products, you'll be eating lots of the protein, fibre and key nutrients that are essential to sustaining muscle mass.

Foods to Avoid

When you eat more healthily, there are foods that you need to cut out. It's the usual suspects: fats should be the healthy kind, so, butter, vegetable shortening and coconut oil are not recommended.

You should also limit the amounts of starchy vegetables you eat: corn, potatoes and peas, etc. Those with a sweet tooth: sugary drinks, desserts, cookies and chocolate are all out.

How Often Do You Eat on Lean and Green Diet?

As you know, it's not what you eat or when you eat that's crucial to weight loss. How often you eat is also an important aspect. Lean and green is no exception to this rule.

The eating habits and preferences that everyone has are as unique as their biology and personality. We are all creatures of habit. Some of our habits are good and some not so good! There are people who enjoy eating at least one large meal every day, but they don't refuel in between times. They start their day with a hearty breakfast, and eat frugally throughout the day. Some skip breakfast altogether, then have a quick snack for lunch, because they prefer to eat their main meal later. Some busy people are "grazers" who like to eat small, frequent meals. There is one group of people who snack all day long, and never eat a balanced meal.

Eating habits, and preferences for certain foods are a totally personal thing. There are carb-loaders, there are sugar cravers, some are into fatty foods, and some are more health-conscious, following plant-based diets. Some people have to adjust their habits when they go Lean and Green.

As I explained, the essence of the Lean and Green diet is to "fuel" your body regularly throughout the day, in order to supplement either one, two or three main meals. The simplicity and versatility of the Lean and Green diet is really helpful. You can try out all three plans, to see which one best meets your needs, and continues to work well for you over time. Once you reach your target weight, you can experiment. The cookbook will help you to do this, because it gives you recipes to prepare when you want to eat balanced, fresh food.

The Lean and Green diet advises that you eat six or seven times per day depending on the plan.

Optimal Weight 5 & 1 Plan

This is the most popular plan, it includes five fuelings, and one balanced Lean and Green meal each day.

Optimal Weight 4 & 2 & 1 Plan

This is for people who need more calories and flexibility in food choices. This includes four fuelings, two Lean and Green meals, and one snack per day.

Optimal Health 3 & 3 Plan is specially designed for maintenance. It includes three fuelings and three balanced Lean and Green meals per day.

How Does Lean and Green Diet Work for Weight Loss?

The Lean and Green diet will work for you and support you if you want to lose excess weight and body fat and maintain the changes. One of the main reasons that the Lean and Green diet does work so efficiently is that the diet plan is so easy to implement and maintain, so you don't "fall off the wagon" and cheat yourself, by eating more than you should or foods that you shouldn't eat. The Lean and Green diet helps you to lose weight and cut your body fat because it is designed very precisely, to help you to quickly get rid of those unwanted extra inches. It helps you to achieve this by reducing the calories and carbs that you eat every day, through the use of the carefully portion-controlled meals and snacks that are included in the program. If you are using these meals and snacks and combining them with a regular exercise regime, (and you are not cheating and snacking on chocolate!) the end result that you achieve will be a substantial overall weight loss, and improved health that you can easily maintain.

Over the last twenty years, weight loss has become an influential industry, with many diets and products on the market. So, necessarily, there has been a lot of clinical research into the efficiency and safety of weight loss products and diets. Some studies have clearly shown that greater weight loss is ensured if those who wish to lose weight follow a regime that contains either full or partial meal replacement plans, compared with more traditional calorie-restricted diets which do not contain any meal replacement products.

The bottom line is that by reducing your overall calorie intake, the Lean and Green diet is going to be very effective for weight loss. If you follow the Lean and Green diet, as per the recommendations, it makes changing your eating habits very easy to do. A comprehensive sixteen-week study of 198 people confirmed that the people who were on the Lean and Green 5 & 1 Plan had significantly lower weight, and body fat, as well as smaller waist circumferences, compared with the people who were in the control group, who were not on the Lean and Green diet. Most people on the 5 & 1 Plan lost 5.7% of their body weight, though 28.1% lost 10%. The same study found that individuals on the 5 & 1 diet who completed at least 75% of the available coaching sessions lost twice as much weight as those who participated less.

Give the Lean and Green diet a try. Using this supporting cookbook, the only thing that you have to lose is weight!

Lean and Green Recipes

Spinach and Egg Breakfast Burrito

1 Leaner | 3 Greens | 1 Healthy Fat | 3 Condiments Prep
time: 10 minutes | Cook time: 10 minutes | Serves 2

Tortillas:

2 tablespoons whole flax seeds

2 eggs

4 egg whites

Filling:

2 cups loosely chopped baby spinach 1 cup
shredded reduced-fat Pepper Jack cheese

Salsa:

1 cup diced tomatoes

½ cup diced bell pepper

1 jalapeño pepper, diced

¼ cup fresh chopped cilantro

1 clove garlic, minced

1 tablespoon chopped red onion

2 teaspoons balsamic vinegar

⅛ teaspoon salt

⅛ teaspoon pepper

1. Whisk together all the tortilla ingredients in a small bowl until combined.

2. Heat a small skillet over medium-high heat and spritz lightly with cooking spray.

3. Pour half of the egg mixture into the hot skillet, swirling to spread the egg mixture evenly on the surface. Cook for 2 minutes until the edges and bottom of the tortilla are firm. Tilt the skillet from side to side to make sure that the eggs are no longer runny. Using a spatula, gently loosen the tortilla from the surface and carefully flip. Continue to cook for an additional 1 to 2 minutes, or until the eggs are completely set. Repeat with the remaining half of the egg mixture. Set the tortillas aside when finished.

4. Lightly spray the skillet with cooking spray again. Add the spinach and sauté for 2 to 3 minutes until wilted, over low to medium-high heat. When done, remove from the heat and set aside.

5. In a medium-sized mixing bowl, combine all the salsa ingredients and stir to incorporate.

6. Arrange the tortillas on two large plates. Divide half of sautéed spinach, cheese, and salsa into the middle of each tortilla, and then roll into a burrito. Serve immediately.

Crab and Asparagus Frittata

1 Leanest | 3 Greens | 2 Healthy Fats | 3 Condiments

Prep time: 8 minutes | Cook time: 30 minutes | Serves 4

2 pounds (907 g) asparagus, woody ends trimmed and cut into bite-sized pieces

2½ tablespoons extra-virgin olive oil, divided

1 teaspoon salt

2 teaspoons sweet paprika

½ teaspoon black pepper

1 pound (454 g) lump crab meat

4 cups liquid egg substitute

¼ cup chopped basil

1 tablespoon finely chopped chives

1. Preheat the oven to 375ºF (190ºC). Line a baking sheet with parchment paper.

2. Toss the asparagus with 2 tablespoons of olive oil, salt, paprika, and black pepper until evenly coated. Spread the asparagus onto the prepared baking sheet. Bake in the preheated oven for about 10 minutes until crisp-tender.

3. Meanwhile, combine the crab meat, liquid egg substitute, basil, and chives in a mixing bowl and stir until well incorporated.

4. Heat the remaining ½ tablespoon of olive oil in an ovenproof skillet over medium heat. Carefully pour the crab mixture into the skillet with the cooked asparagus, and gently stir to mix well. Cook until the eggs start to bubble.

5. Put the skillet in the oven and bake, or until the eggs are completely cooked and golden brown, about 15 to 20 minutes.

6. Cool for 5 minutes and serve.

Zucchini and Spinach Manicotti

1 Lean | 3 Greens | 1 Condiment

Prep time: 10 minutes | Cook time: 25 minutes | Serves 4

1 ½ cups part-skim ricotta cheese

1 cup frozen spinach, thawed and patted dry

1 ½ cups reduced-fat shredded Mozzarella cheese, divided

1 egg, lightly beaten

¼ cup grated Parmesan cheese

⅛ teaspoon salt

Pinch nutmeg

2 large zucchinis, sliced into ⅛-inch-thick slices

1 cup low-sugar tomato sauce

1. Preheat the oven to 375ºF (190ºC).

2. Mix together the ricotta, spinach, ½ cup of Mozzarella, beaten egg, Parmesan, salt, and nutmeg in a medium mixing bowl and stir to combine.

3. On a clean work surface, layer three slices of zucchini parallel to each other. Place a large spoonful of ricotta mixture on one end of the zucchini slices and roll up. Arrange the stuffed zucchini in a lightly greased baking dish. Pour the tomato sauce over top of the zucchini and scatter with the remaining 1 cup of Mozzarella.

4. Bake in the preheated oven for 25 minutes until the cheese melts.

5. Remove from the oven and rest for 5 minutes before serving.

Pork and Green Tomatillo Stew

1 Lean | 3 Greens | 3 Condiments

Prep time: 15 minutes | Cook time: 20 minutes | Serves 4

1 pound (454 g) tomatillos, trimmed and chopped

8 large romaine or green lettuce leaves, divided

2 serrano chilies, seeds and membranes removed, chopped

2 scallions, chopped

2 cloves garlic

½ teaspoon dried oregano

1 ½ pounds (680 g) boneless pork loin, cut into bite-sized cubes

¼ teaspoon salt

¼ teaspoon pepper

1 cup sliced radishes

¼ cup chopped cilantro

1 jalapeño, seeds and membranes removed, thinly sliced

4 lime wedges

1. Place the tomatillos, 4 lettuce leaves, serrano chilies, scallions, garlic, and oregano in a blender and purée until smooth.

2. Add the pork and tomatillo mixture into a medium pot (the pork should be covered by 1-inch of tomatillo mixture; if not, add the water until it is). Sprinkle with the salt and pepper. Cover and bring to a simmer over low heat, about 20 minutes.

3. Meanwhile, finely shred the remaining 4 lettuce leaves.

4. Garnish the stew with the radishes, cilantro, shredded lettuce, jalapeño slices, and lime wedges, then serve.

BBQ Pork with Greek Yogurt Slaw

1 Lean | 3 Greens | 3 Condiments

Prep time: 10 minutes | Cook time: 1 hour 10 minutes | Serves 4

1(1 ½ pounds / 680 g) pork tenderloin, cut in half

Cooking spray

1 (12-ounce / 340-g) can diet root

beer ½ cup sugar- free barbecue

sauce **Slaw:**

3 cups shredded red cabbage

3 cups shredded green cabbage

½ cup low-fat plain Greek yogurt

1 tablespoon apple cider vinegar

1 teaspoon Dijon mustard

2 teaspoons lemon juice

¼ teaspoon celery salt

Pinch stevia

1. Grease the bottom of the Instant Pot with cooking spray. Set the Instant Pot to Sauté and brown the pork on all sides, about 3 minutes per side.

2. Pour in the beer and mix well.

3. Secure the lid. Select the Manual mode and set the cooking time for 60 minutes at High Pressure.

4. Meanwhile, stir together all the slaw ingredients in a medium bowl until combined. Set aside.

5. When the timer beeps, perform a natural pressure release for 10 minutes, then release any remaining pressure. Carefully remove the lid.

6. Transfer the pork to a large bowl and shred the meat. Add the barbecue sauce and toss well. Serve the pulled pork with the slaw on the side.

Baked Pork Chops with Vegetables

1 Lean | 3 Greens | 3 Condiments

Prep time: 5 to 10 minutes | Cook time: 28 minutes | Serves 4

1 ½ pounds (680 g) boneless pork chops

½ teaspoon salt, divided

¼ teaspoon pepper, divided

1 teaspoon dried thyme

Cooking spray

¼ cup low-sodium chicken broth

1 (8-ounce / 227-g) package sliced baby bella mushrooms

4 cloves garlic, minced

⅛ teaspoon crushed red pepper flakes

2 (10-ounce / 283-g) bags Swiss or rainbow chard, sliced and washed

¼ cup freshly grated Parmesan cheese

1. Preheat the oven to 450ºF (235ºC).

2. Season pork chops with ¼ teaspoon of salt, ⅛ teaspoon of pepper, and thyme.

3. Lightly grease a large skillet and heat over medium high heat. Add the chops and light brown each side for 3 to 4 minutes. Remove from heat and set aside.

4. Pour the chicken broth into the same skillet. Sauté mushrooms with garlic and red pepper flakes until just tender.

5. Arrange the chard in a large casserole dish, and season with remaining salt and pepper. Add mushroom mixture and the pork chops. Sprinkle with the Parmesan cheese.

6. Bake in the preheated oven for 18 to 20 minutes, or until the internal temperature of pork reaches 145ºF (63ºC).

7. Serve warm.

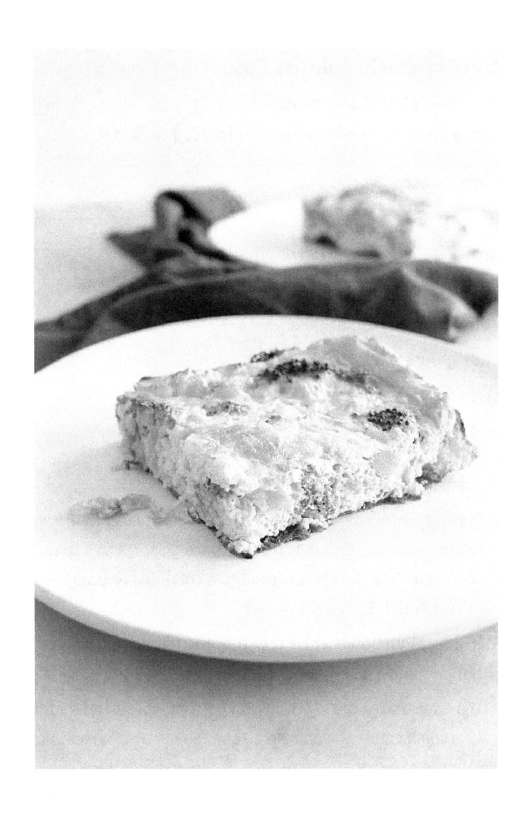

Broccoli Cheese Breakfast Casserole

1 Lean | 3 Greens | 1½ Condiments

Prep time: 5 minutes | Cook time: 45 minutes | Serves 4

6 cups small broccoli florets

9 eggs

1 cup unsweetened almond milk

¼ teaspoon salt

¼ teaspoon cayenne pepper

¼ teaspoon ground pepper

Cooking spray

4 ounces (113 g) shredded, reduced-fat Cheddar cheese

1. Preheat the oven to 375ºF (190ºC).

2. Place the broccoli with 2 to 3 tablespoons water in a large microwave-safe dish. Microwave on High for 3 to 4 minutes or until softened. Transfer the broccoli to a colander to drain off any excess liquid. Set aside.

3. In a medium bowl, whisk together the eggs, milk, salt, cayenne pepper, and ground pepper to combine.

4. Lightly grease a baking dish with cooking spray and add the broccoli. Scatter the cheese all over the broccoli, then pour the egg mixture over top.

5. Bake in the preheated oven for 40 to 45 minutes, or until a toothpick inserted into the center comes out clean and the top is lightly browned.

6. Let rest for 5 minutes before slicing and serving.

Bibimbap Bowls

1 Leaner | 3 Greens | 1 Healthy Fat | 2 Condiments
Prep time: 10 minutes | Cook time: 12 minutes | Serves 4

1 teaspoon olive oil

5 cups baby spinach

1 teaspoon toasted sesame oil

¼ teaspoon salt

1 pound (454 g) 95 to 97% lean ground beef

1 tablespoon reduced-sodium soy sauce

2 tablespoons chili garlic sauce

2 cups riced cauliflower

1 cup thinly sliced cucumber

4 hard-boiled eggs

½ cup chopped green onions

1 tablespoon sesame seeds

1. Heat the olive oil in a skillet over medium high heat until it shimmers. Add the baby spinach and sauté for 2 to 3 minutes until just wilted. Drizzle with the sesame oil and season with salt.

2. Remove the spinach from the skillet and set aside.

3. Place the ground beef in the same skillet and cook until fully browned. Stir in the chili garlic sauce and soy sauce and cook for 1 minute. Remove the skillet from the heat and set aside.

4. Place the riced cauliflower with 1 tablespoon water in a large microwave-safe dish. Microwave on High for 3 to 4 minutes or until tender.

5. Divide ½ cup of riced cauliflower into each bowl. Top each bowl evenly with the spinach, beef, and sliced cucumber. Place an egg on top of each bowl. Serve garnished with the green onions and green onions.

Mini Bacon Cheeseburger Bites

1 Lean | 1 Green | 3 Condiments

Prep time: 10 minutes | Cook time: 18 minutes | Serves 4

1 pound (454 g) lean ground beef

¼ cup finely chopped yellow onion

1 tablespoon Worcestershire sauce

1 tablespoon yellow mustard

1 clove garlic, minced

½ teaspoon salt

Cooking spray

4 ultra-thin slices Cheddar cheese, each cut into 6 equal-sized rectangular pieces

3 pieces cooked turkey bacon, each cut into 8 equal-sized rectangular pieces

24 dill pickle chips

4 to 6 large green leaf lettuce leaves, torn into 24 (total) small squareshaped pieces

12 cherry tomatoes, sliced in half

1. Preheat the oven to 400ºF (205ºC). Line a baking sheet with aluminum foil.

2. In a medium mixing bowl, stir together the ground beef, onion, Worcestershire sauce, mustard, garlic, and salt until well mixed. Shape the mixture into 24 small meatballs. Arrange the meatballs on the prepared baking sheet and spray them with cooking spray.

3. Bake in the preheated oven for about 15 minutes until cooked through.

4. Place a piece of cheese on top of each meatball and bake for an additional 2 to 3 minutes, or until the cheese is melted. Remove from the oven and let cool.

5. Assemble the bites: On a toothpick, layer a cheese -covered meatball, piece of bacon, pickle chip, piece of lettuce, and cherry tomato half, in that order. Serve immediately.

Mongolian Beef

1 Lean | 3 Greens | 2½ Condiments

Prep time: 10 minutes | Cook time: 15 minutes | Serves 4

4 cups cauliflower rice

Cooking spray

1 ½ pounds (680 g) flank steak, thinly sliced

2 cups broccoli florets

½ cup chicken or beef broth

1 cup diced scallions

$1/3$ cup reduced sodium soy sauce

1 teaspoon minced fresh ginger

2 cloves garlic, minced

½ teaspoon red pepper flakes

1. Heat a lightly greased skillet over medium-high heat. Add the cauliflower rice and cook for about 3 to 5 minutes, until tender. Remove the cauliflower rice from the skillet and set aside.

2. Lightly grease the skillet with cooking spray and add the beef. Cook over medium-high heat for about 4 to 5 minutes until cooked through, flipping the slices halfway through.

3. Add the broccoli and broth to the skillet with the beef. Continue to cook until the broccoli turns bright green and just softened.

4. Add the remaining ingredients to the skillet and stir to combine. Cook for an additional 1 to 2 minutes.

5. Remove from the heat and serve over cauliflower rice.

Cheesy Cod with Tomatoes

1 Leanest | 3 Greens | 2 Healthy Fats | 3 Condiments
Prep time: 15 minutes | Cook time: 40 minutes | Serves 4

2 garlic cloves

4 scallions, chopped with green and white parts separated

2 ½ tablespoons olive oil, divided

2 ½ cups diced canned tomatoes, with their juice

¼ teaspoon dried oregano

3 small zucchinis (about 12 ounces / 340 g), sliced lengthwise into ⅛-inchthick slices

1 ¾ pounds (794 g) cod fillets, cut into 12 equal-sized pieces

½ teaspoon kosher salt

½ teaspoon ground black pepper, divided

⅓ cup reduced-fat crumbled feta cheese

1 cup chopped fresh whole basil leaves

1. In a saucepan, cook the garlic and white parts of scallions in 1 tablespoon of olive oil until fragrant, about 2 minutes.

2. Add the tomatoes with their juice and oregano. Bring to a gentle simmer for 20 minutes or until thickened.

3. Remove from the heat and stir in the green parts of scallions. Set aside.

4. Preheat the oven to 425ºF (220ºC).

5. Lay the zucchini slices in an ovenproof casserole dish and top with the cod fillets. Sprinkle with the salt and ¼ teaspoon of black

pepper. Drizzle with the remaining olive oil. Scatter the cooked tomatoes and feta cheese on top.

6. Bake in the preheated oven for 20 minutes, or until the cod reaches an internal temperature of 145ºF (63ºC).

7. Serve topped with the basil leaves and remaining ¼ teaspoon of black pepper.

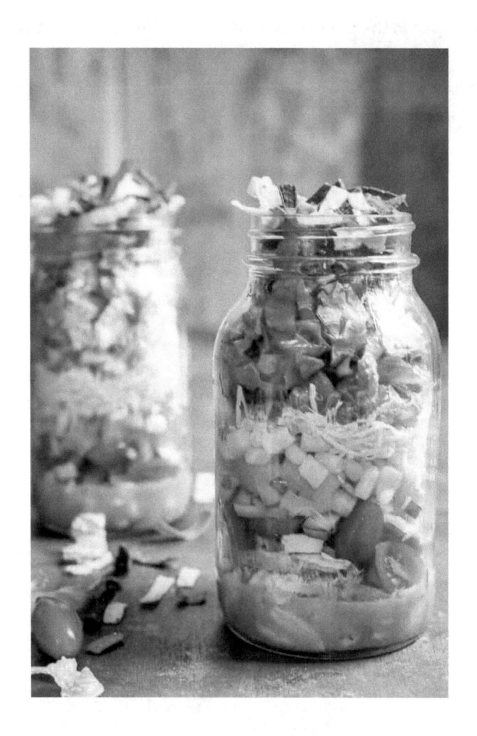

Taco Mason Jar Salad

1 Lean | 3 Greens | 3 Condiments

Prep time: 15 minutes | Cook time: 10 minutes | Serves 2

Beef:

½ pound (227 g) 90 to 94% lean ground beef

½ tablespoon taco seasoning **Dressing:**

½ cup loosely packed fresh cilantro

⅓ cup nonfat plain Greek yogurt

Juice of half a lime

1 clove garlic

Pinch salt **Salad:**

½ cup Pico de Gallo (see below)

½ cup reduced-fat Mexican blend shredded cheese

1 medium-sized bell pepper,

diced 3 cups shredded lettuce

Pico de Gallo:

1 tomato, diced

½ large white onion, diced

½ jalapeño pepper, stemmed, seeded, and diced

2 tablespoons chopped fresh cilantro

1 tablespoon freshly squeezed lime juice

⅛ teaspoon salt

Make the Pico de Gallo

1. Mix together the tomato, onion, pepper, cilantro, lime juice, and salt in a bowl. Stir well with a fork to incorporate. Set aside.

Make the Salad

2. Heat a medium skillet over medium-high heat. Add the beef and sprinkle with the taco seasoning, and cook until the beef is browned, stirring occasionally.

3. Meanwhile, combine the cilantro, yogurt, lime juice, garlic, and salt in a blender and purée until smooth.

4. Assemble the mason jar salads: Evenly divide each salad ingredient among two mason jars and layer in the following order: dressing, pico de gallo, beef, cheese, bell pepper, and shredded lettuce.
Cover and refrigerate until ready to eat.

Lemon Pepper Salmon with Parmesan Asparagus

1 Lean | 3 Greens | 3 Condiments

Prep time: 5 minutes | Cook time: 15 to 20 minutes | Serves 4

1 ½ pounds (680 g) salmon, skin-on

Cooking spray

2 teaspoons salt-free lemon pepper seasoning

½ teaspoon salt

Lemon slices, for garnish

¼ cup grated Parmesan cheese

½ teaspoon garlic powder

1 ½ pounds (680 g) asparagus, woody ends trimmed

1. Preheat the oven to 400ºF (205ºC). Line a baking sheet with aluminum foil and spray it with cooking spray.

2. Put the salmon in the center of baking sheet and spritz the salmon lightly with cooking spray. Sprinkle with the lemon pepper seasoning and salt. Scatter the lemon slices on top.

3. Combine the Parmesan cheese and garlic powder in a small bowl. Arrange the asparagus spears around the salmon. Lightly spritz with cooking spray and scatter with the Parmesan cheese mixture.

4. Bake in the preheated oven for about 15 to 20 minutes, or until the salmon is cooked through.

5. Serve hot.

Easy Salmon Florentine

1 Lean | 3 Greens | 3 Condiments

Prep time: 15 minutes | Cook time: 20 minutes | Serves 4

½ cup chopped green onions

1 teaspoon olive oil

2 garlic cloves, minced

1 (12-ounce / 340-g) package frozen chopped spinach, thawed and patted dry

1 ½ cups chopped cherry tomatoes

¼ teaspoon crushed red pepper flakes

¼ teaspoon pepper

¼ teaspoon salt

½ cup part-skim ricotta cheese

4 (5½-ounce / 156-g) wild salmon fillets

Cooking spray

1. Preheat the oven to 350ºF (180ºC).

2. In a medium skillet, cook the onions in the olive oil for about 2 minutes, or until they begin to soften.

3. Add the minced garlic and cook for another 1 minute. Add the spinach, tomatoes, red pepper flakes, pepper and salt. Cook, stirring, for 2 minutes.

4. Remove from heat and let cool for 10 minutes. Stir in the ricotta cheese.

5. Put a quarter of the spinach mixture on top of each salmon fillet. Arrange the fillets on a lightly greased rimmed baking sheet. Bake

in the preheated oven until the salmon is cooked through, for 15 minutes.

6. Cool for 5 minutes before serving.

Cilantro Salmon with Bell Peppers

1 Lean | 3 Greens | 3 Condiments

Prep time: 15 minutes | Cook time: 32 minutes | Serves 4

4 cups fresh cilantro, divided

2 tablespoons fresh lemon juice

2 tablespoons hot red pepper sauce

1 teaspoon cumin

½ teaspoon salt, divided

½ cup water

4 (7-ounce / 198-g) raw salmon fillets

2 cups sliced red bell pepper

2 cups sliced green bell pepper

2 cups sliced yellow bell pepper

½ teaspoon ground black pepper

Cooking spray

1. In a food processor, combine half of the cilantro, lemon juice, hot red pepper sauce, cumin, ¼ teaspoon of salt, and water. Pulse until creamy. Transfer the marinade to a resealable plastic bag.

2. Dunk the salmon into the marinade. Seal the bag and shake to make sure the salmon is coated well.

3. Put the bag in the refrigerator. Refrigerate for an hour, turning bag occasionally.

4. Preheat the oven to 400ºF (205ºC).

5. Arrange the pepper slices in a greased baking dish. Sprinkle with black pepper and remaining salt.

6. Bake in the preheated oven for 20 minutes, flipping the pepper slices once.

7. Remove the bag from the refrigerator. Discard the marinade. Dust the salmon with remaining cilantro.

8. Place salmon on top of pepper slices, and bake for an additional 12 minutes or until tender.

9. Serve immediately.

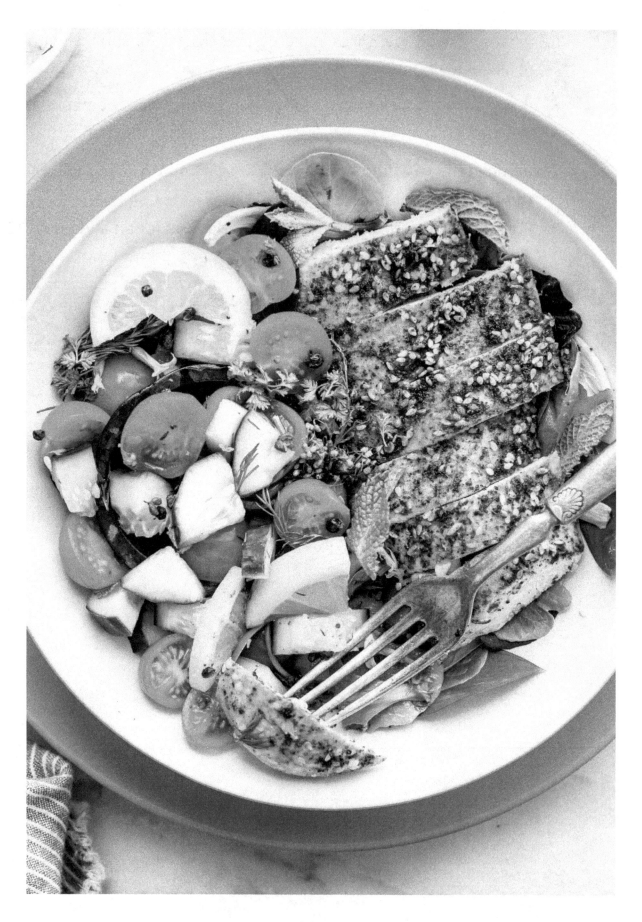

Za'atar Salmon with Cucumber Salad

1 Lean | 3 Greens | 3 Condiments

Prep time: 5 minutes | Cook time: 25 minutes | Serves 4

Salad:

4 cups sliced cucumber

1 pint cherry tomatoes, halved

¼ cup chopped fresh dill

¼ cup cider vinegar

¼ teaspoon salt ¼

teaspoon black pepper

Salmon:

1 ½ pounds (680 g) skinless salmon

1 tablespoon Za'atar

4 lemon wedges

1. Preheat the oven to 350ºF (180ºC). Line a baking sheet with aluminum foil.

2. Toss all the salad ingredients in a bowl until combined. Set aside.

3. Season the salmon with Za'atar on both sides, and place on the prepared baking sheet.

4. Roast in the preheated oven for about 25 minutes, or until the internal temperature registers 145ºF (63ºC).

5. Serve the salmon with the salad and lemon wedges.

Shrimp and Creamy Cauliflower Grits

1 Leanest | 3 Greens | 2 Healthy Fats | 3 Condiments
Prep time: 10 minutes | Cook time: 15 minutes | Serves 2

1 pound (454 g) raw, peeled and deveined shrimp

½ tablespoon Cajun seasoning

Cooking spray

¼ cup chicken broth

1 tablespoon lemon juice

1 tablespoon butter

2 ½ cups finely riced cauliflower

½ cup unsweetened almond or cashew milk

¼ teaspoon salt

$1/3$ cup reduced-fat shredded Cheddar cheese

2 tablespoons sour cream

¼ cup thinly sliced scallions

1. Add the shrimp and Cajun seasoning into a large, resealable plastic bag. Seal the bag and toss to coat well.

2. Grease a skillet with cooking spray and heat over medium heat.

3. Add the shrimp and cook each side for about 2 to 3 minutes. Add chicken broth and lemon juice, scraping any bits off of the bottom of the pan, and let simmer for 1 minute. Remove from the heat and set aside.

4. In a separate skillet, melt the butter over medium heat.

5. Add the riced cauliflower and cook for 5 minutes. Add milk and salt and cook for an additional 5 minutes.

6. Remove from heat and stir in sour cream and cheese until melted.

7. Serve the shrimp over cauliflower grits and sprinkle with the scallions.

Shrimp Scampi with Zucchini Noodles

1 Leanest | 3 Greens | 2 Healthy Fats | 3 Condiments
Prep time: 10 minutes | Cook time: 10 minutes | Serves 2

1 tablespoon butter

2 teaspoons olive oil

2 cloves garlic, minced

1 ½ pounds (680 g) raw shrimp, peeled, and deveined

½ teaspoon crushed red pepper flakes

¼ cup chicken broth

1 tablespoon lemon juice

½ teaspoon lemon zest

¼ teaspoon salt

3 small zucchini, spiralized

1. Heat the butter and olive oil in a large skillet over medium heat.
2. Add the garlic, shrimp, and crushed red pepper flakes. Cook for about 3 to 5 minutes, stirring occasionally, or until shrimp are pink.
3. Stir in chicken broth, lemon juice, and lemon zest. Sprinkle with the salt. Bring to a simmer. Add the zucchini noodles and stir to combine, about 1 to 2 minutes. Serve warm.

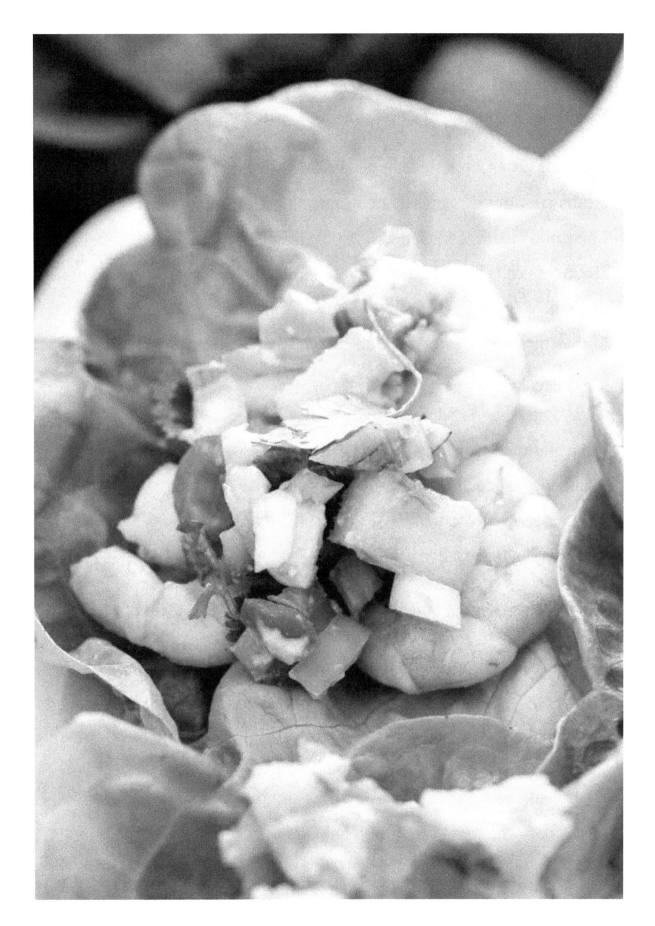

Shrimp and Avocado Lettuce Wraps

1 Leanest | 3 Greens | 2 Healthy Fats | 3 Condiments
Prep time: 15 minutes | Cook time: 6 minutes | Serves 4

2 pounds (907 g) raw shrimp, peeled and deveined

1 tablespoon Old Bay blackened seasoning

4 teaspoons olive oil, divided

6 ounces (170 g) avocado

1 cup plain Greek yogurt

2 tablespoons lime juice, divided

1 ½ cups diced tomato

¼ cup diced green bell pepper

¼ cup chopped cilantro

1 jalapeño pepper, chopped and deseeded

¼ cup chopped red onion

12 large romaine lettuce leaves

1. Place shrimp and Old Bay seasoning in a resealable plastic bag. Shake to coat well.

2. Heat 2 teaspoons of olive oil in a skillet and add the shrimp. Cook for 5 minutes on both sides or until shrimp are pink and cooked through. You may need to work in batches to avoid overcrowding.

3. Combine the avocado, Greek yogurt, and 1 tablespoon of lime juice in a food processor. Pulse until smooth.

4. Stir the tomatoes, green bell pepper, cilantro, jalapeño pepper, onion, and remaining tablespoon of lime juice in a medium bowl.

5. Divide the shrimp, avocado mixture, and tomato mixture among the lettuce leaves.

6. Serve immediately.

Seared Scallops over Zucchini Noodles

1 Leanest | 3 Greens | 2 Healthy Fats | 2 Condiments
Prep time: 10 minutes | Cook time: 15 minutes | Serves 2

2 small zucchinis, ends removed, and spiralized

½ tablespoon butter

1 pound (454 g) raw
scallops ⅛ teaspoon salt

Sauce:

6 ounces (170 g) jarred roasted red peppers, drained

2 ounces (57 g) avocado

½ cup unsweetened almond or cashew milk

2 teaspoons lemon juice

1 clove garlic

¼ teaspoon salt

¼ teaspoon crushed red pepper (optional)

1. Combine all the sauce ingredients in a blender and purée until smooth.

2. Heat the roasted red pepper sauce in a skillet over medium heat, stirring occasionally, until heated through, about 3 to 5 minutes.

3. Stir in the zucchini noodles and continue to cook for an additional 3 to 5 minutes, or until cooked to your preference.

4. Meanwhile, melt the butter in a large skillet over medium-high heat. Season the scallops with salt. Cook the scallops until golden brown on each side and translucent in the center, about 1 to 2 minutes per side.

5. Serve the scallops over the zucchini noodles.

Lemon Garlic Chicken Thighs with Asparagus

1 Lean| 3 Greens | 2 Condiments

Prep time: 5 minutes | Cook time: 40 minutes | Serves 4

1 ¾ pounds (794 g) bone-in, skinless chicken thighs

2 tablespoons lemon juice

2 tablespoons minced fresh oregano

2 cloves garlic, minced

¼ teaspoon pepper

¼ teaspoon salt

2 pounds (907 g) asparagus, trimmed

1. Preheat the oven to 350ºF (180ºC).
2. Toss all the ingredients except the asparagus in a mixing bowl until combined.
3. Roast the chicken thighs in the preheated oven for about 40 minutes, or until it reaches an internal temperature of 165ºF (74ºC).
4. When cooked, remove the chicken thighs from the oven and set aside to cool.
5. Meanwhile, steam the asparagus in the microwave to the desired doneness.
6. Serve the asparagus with roasted chicken thighs.

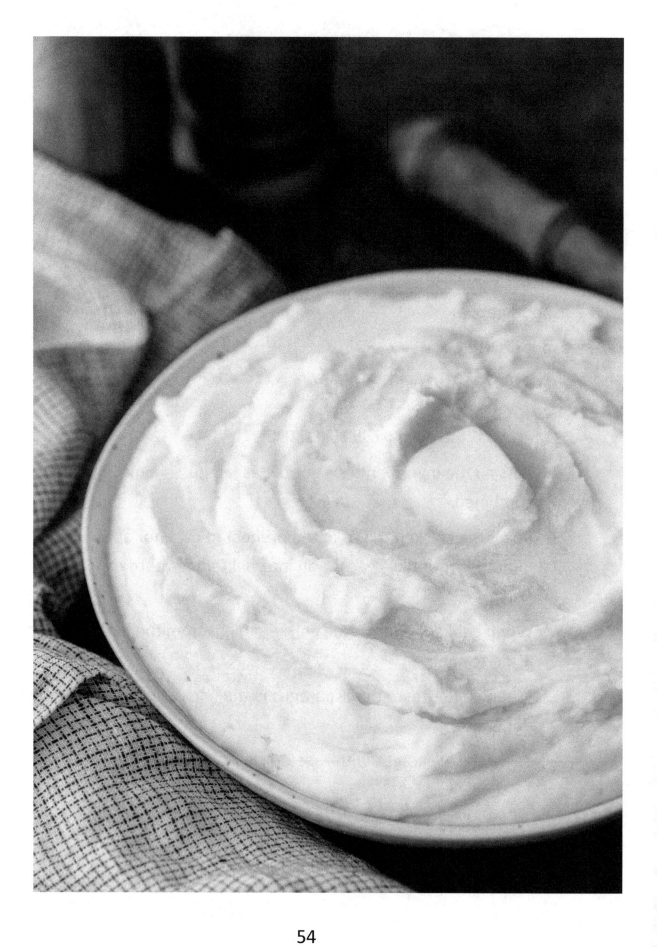

Fueling Hacks

Cheesy Smashed Potato

1 Fueling | ½ Leaner

Prep time: 5 minutes | Cook time: 12 minutes | Serves 2

2 sachets Optavia Essential Smashed Potatoes

1 cup water

1 cup reduced fat, shredded Mozzarella cheese

1. In a microwave-safe bowl, mix the Optavia Essential Smashed Potatoes and water to combine well.

2. Microwave on high for 1½ minutes, then stir.

3. Pour the mixture into a lightly greased waffle iron. Close lid and cook for 10 minutes or until lightly browned.

4. Open the lid and sprinkle with the cheese on one half of the waffle. Fold over the other half of the waffle.

5. Close the lid and continue cooking for 2 minutes or until cheese melts.

6. Serve immediately.

Easy Avocado Toast

1 Fueling | 1 Healthy Fat

Prep time: 5 minutes | Cook time: 15 minutes | Serves 1

1 sachet Optavia Select Buttermilk Cheddar Herb Biscuit

1 ½ ounces (43 g) avocado, mashed

1. Bake the Buttermilk Cheddar Herb Biscuit according to the package directions.
2. Allow to cool before serving with mashed avocado on top.

Simple Yogurt Chocolate Cookie Dough

1 Fueling | ½ Leaner

Prep time: 5 minutes | Cook time: 0 minutes | Serves 1

1 sachet Optavia Essential Chewy Chocolate Chip Cookie

1 (5.3-ounce / 150-g) container low-fat plain Greek yogurt

1. Combine the Chewy Chocolate Chip Cookie with the Greek yogurt in a bowl.

2. Chill until ready to serve.

Cinnamon Oatmeal Bake with Pecans

1 Fueling | 1 Healthy Fat | 1 Condiment

Prep time: 10 minutes | Cook time: 20 to 25 minutes | Serves 4

4 sachets Optavia Indonesian Cinnamon and Honey Hot Cereal

½ teaspoon baking powder

1 cup unsweetened almond milk

3 tablespoons egg whites

1 ½ ounces (43 g) chopped pecans

¼ teaspoon cinnamon

Cooking spray

Special Equipment:

4 (4.2-ounce / 125-ml) mini mason jars

1. Preheat the oven to 350ºF (180ºC).

2. Combine the Indonesian Cinnamon and Honey Hot Cereal and baking powder in a bowl. Stir in the almond milk and egg white. Fold in the pecans.

3. Spritz 4 mason jars with cooking spray. Divide the mixture evenly between the jars, leaving 2 inches at the top. Sprinkle with cinnamon.

4. Bake in the preheated oven for 20 to 25 minutes on a baking sheet or until golden.

5. Allow to cool. Close the lid, refrigerate, and serve chilled.

Cheese and Tomato Caprese Pizza Bites

1 Fueling | ¼ Lean | ½ Green | ½ Healthy Fat | 2 Condiments Prep
time: 10 minutes | Cook time: 12 minutes | Serves 4

4 sachets Optavia Buttermilk Cheddar Herb Biscuit

½ cup unsweetened almond milk

2 teaspoons olive oil

1 cup basil leaves, julienned

4 ounces (113 g) fresh Mozzarella log, cut into 12 small pieces

3 Roma tomatoes, thinly sliced

2 tablespoons balsamic vinegar

Cooking spray

1. Preheat the oven to 450ºF (235ºC).

2. In a bowl, mix Buttermilk Cheddar Herb Biscuit, almond milk, and olive oil until well combined.

3. Divide the biscuit mixture among 12 slots of a greased muffin tin.

4. Layer a slice of Mozzarella, then a slice of tomato, and then a few pieces of basil into each slot.

5. Bake in the preheated oven for 12 minutes or until biscuit mixture is well browned and cheese is bubbly.

6. Drizzle with balsamic vinegar on top before serving.

Creamy Yogurt Berry Bagels

1 Fueling | ½ Healthy Fat | 1½ Condiments

Prep time: 10 minutes | Cook time: 15 minutes | Serves 2

2 sachets Optavia Essential Yogurt Berry Blast Smoothie

2 tablespoons liquid egg substitute

$1/3$ cup unsweetened almond milk

½ teaspoon baking powder

Cooking spray

1 ounce (28 g) light cream cheese

1. Preheat the oven to 350ºF (180ºC).

2. In a bowl, mix the Yogurt Berry Blast Smoothie with egg substitute, almond milk, and baking powder.

3. Divide mixture among 4 greased slots of a donut pan.

4. Bake in the preheated oven for 15 minutes or until set.

5. Spread the cream cheese on top and allow to cool before serving.

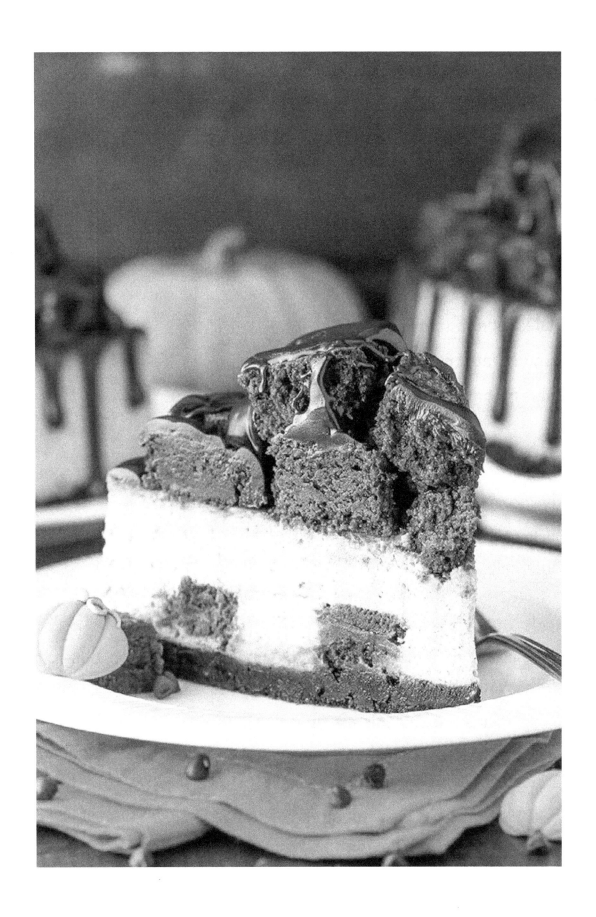

Chocolate Pumpkin Cheesecake

1 Fueling | ½ Leaner | 1 Healthy Fat | 3 Condiments
Prep time: 15 minutes | Cook time: 50 minutes | Serves 1

2 sachets Optavia Essential Decadent Double Chocolate Brownie

½ tablespoon unsalted butter, melted

2 tablespoons water

Cooking spray

3 tablespoons pumpkin purée

1 cup nonfat plain Greek yogurt

3 tablespoons light cream cheese, softened

1 egg

½ teaspoon pumpkin pie spice

½ teaspoon vanilla extract

2 packets stevia

   Pinch salt

1. Preheat the oven to 350ºF (180ºC).
2. Combine the Decadent Double Chocolate Brownies, butter, and water in a small bowl.
3. Divide brownie mixture among 2 greased mini springform pans. Press brownie mixture into the bottom. Bake in the preheated oven for 15 minutes.
4. Meanwhile, whisk together the remaining ingredients in a bowl. Divide the mixture among two springform pans.

5. Lower the oven temperature to 300ºF (150ºC). Bake the cheesecakes for 35 minutes or until lightly browned.

6. Allow to cool before serving.

Tropical Macadamia Smoothie Bowl

1 Fueling | 2 Healthy Fats | 2½ Condiments

Prep time: 10 minutes | Cook time: 0 minutes | Serves 1

1 sachet Optavia Essential Tropical Fruit Smoothie

½ cup unsweetened coconut milk

½ cup ice

1 tablespoon shredded, unsweetened coconut

½ ounce (14 g) macadamias, chopped

½ teaspoon lime zest

½ tablespoon chia seeds

1. Add the Tropical Fruit Smoothie, coconut milk, and ice to a blender. Pulse until smooth.

2. Pour the smoothie into a bowl. Spread the remaining ingredients on top and serve.

Spinach and Cracker Stuffed Mushroom

1 Fueling | ½ Healthy Fat | 1 Condiment | 1 Optional Snack Prep
time: 15 minutes | Cook time: 25 minutes | Serves 4

4 sachets Optavia Spinach Pesto Mac and Cheese

2 cups raw spinach, torn into small pieces

¼ cup fresh basil, torn into small pieces

8 ounces (227 g) water

2 packages (10- to 12-ounce / 283- to 340-g) baby bella mushrooms, rinsed
and stems removed

2 sachets Rosemary Sea Salt Crackers, finely crushed

2 tablespoons grated Pecorino Romano cheese

2 teaspoons olive oil

Cooking spray

1. Preheat the oven to 350ºF (180ºC).

2. In a microwave-safe bowl, mix the Spinach Pesto Mac and Cheese,
   spinach, basil, and water until well combined.

3. Microwave on high for 1½ minutes. Stir and let stand for 1 minute.
   Microwave on high for an additional minute. Stir and let sit.

4. Meanwhile, in a small bowl, combine the Rosemary Sea Salt
   Crackers, cheese, and olive oil.

5. Arrange the baby bella mushroom caps, cavity-side up, onto a
   greased and foil-lined baking sheet.

6. Fill each cavity with Mac and Cheese mixture. Top with Cracker
   mixture and press to secure.

7. Bake in the preheated oven for 22 minutes or until lightly browned.

8. Serve immediately.

Pumpkin Gingerbread Latte

1 Fueling | 2½ Condiments

Prep time: 5 minutes | Cook time: 1 minutes | Serves 1

2 tablespoons pumpkin purée

½ cup unsweetened almond milk

1 sachet Optavia Essential Spiced Gingerbread

½ cup strong brewed coffee

1. Combine the pumpkin purée and milk in a microwave-safe mug. Microwave for 1 minute and stir.

2. Mix in the coffee and Spiced Gingerbread. Serve immediately.

Quick Mint Cookies

1 Fueling | 1 Condiment

Prep time: 10 minutes | Cook time: 15 minutes | Serves 4

2 sachets Optavia Essential Decadent Double Chocolate Brownie

2 Optavia Essential Chocolate Mint Cookie Crisp Bars, softened

2 tablespoons unsweetened almond milk

1 tablespoon liquid egg substitute

¼ teaspoon mint extract

1. Preheat the oven to 350ºF (180ºC).

2. In a small bowl, whisk together the Decadent Double Chocolate Brownies, almond milk, egg substitute, and mint extract. Stir in the microwave crunch bars until the bars break into tiny pieces.

3. Form the mixture into eight cookie, then arrange the cookies on a parchment-lined baking sheet

4. Bake in the preheated oven for 15 minutes or until set and lightly browned.

5. Serve immediately.

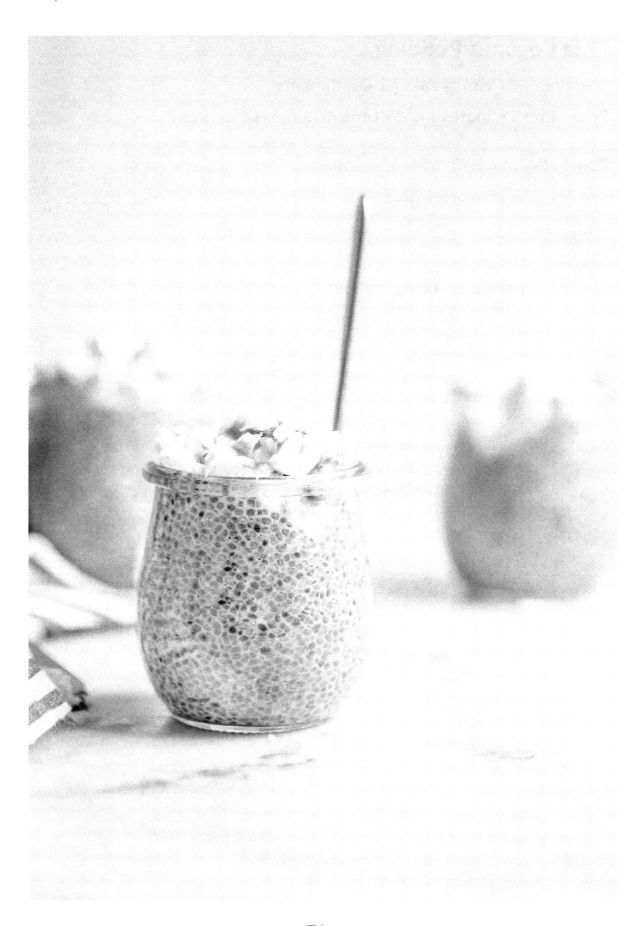

Chia Coconut Pudding

1 Fueling | 2 Healthy Fats | 2 Condiments

Prep time: 5 minutes | Cook time: 0 minutes | Serves 2

2 sachets Optavia Chia Bliss Smoothie

1 cup unsweetened coconut milk

¼ cup chia seeds

1. Combine all the ingredients in a bowl. Stir to mix well.
2. Pour the mixture into a jar and refrigerate overnight.
3. Serve chilled.

Turkey Bacon Savory Potato Waffles

1 Fueling | ½ Lean | 1 Condiments

Prep time: 10 minutes | Cook time: 6 minutes | Serves 4

4 sachets Optavia Essential Roasted Garlic Creamy Smashed Potatoes

½ cup unsweetened almond milk

½ cup shredded, reduced-fat Cheddar cheese

½ cup liquid egg substitute

2 slices turkey bacon, cooked and chopped into small pieces

¼ cup chopped scallions

Cooking spray

1. Mix the Garlic Creamy Smashed Potatoes, almond milk, Cheddar cheese, and egg substitute in a bowl, then stir in the remaining ingredients.

2. Pour the mixture on a greased waffle iron. Close the lid and bake for 6 minutes or until lightly browned.

3. Serve immediately.

Golden Nuggets with Yogurt Dip

1 Fueling | 1 Leaner | 2 Condiments

Prep time: 10 minutes | Cook time: 18 minutes | Serves 2

12 ounces (340 g) boneless, skinless chicken breast, cubed

2 sachets Optavia Essential Honey Mustard and Onion Sticks, crushed into breadcrumb-like consistency

1 egg

¼ cup plain, low-fat Greek yogurt

2 teaspoons spicy brown mustard

¼ teaspoon garlic powder

Cooking Spray

1. Preheat the oven to 400ºF (205ºC).

2. Pour the crushed Honey Mustard and Onion Sticks in a shallow dish, whisk the egg in another bowl.

3. Dredge the chicken cubes into the egg, and then roll over the crushed Honey Mustard and Onion Sticks until coated. Shake the excess off.

4. Place the chicken cubes on a greased, foil-lined baking sheet. Spritz with cooking spray.

5. Bake in the preheated oven for 18 minutes or until the internal temperature reaches at least 165ºF (74ºC), flipping halfway through.

6. Meanwhile, to make the yogurt dip, combine the Greek yogurt, mustard, and garlic powder in a small bowl.

7. Serve the chicken nuggets with yogurt dip.

Rum and Ale Coconut Colada

½ Fueling | 3 Condiments

Prep time: 10 minutes | Cook time: 0 minutes | Serves 1

1 sachet Optavia Essential Creamy Vanilla Shake

6 ounces (170 g) unsweetened, original coconut milk

¼ teaspoon rum extract

6 ounces (170 g) diet ginger ale

½ cup ice

2 tablespoons shredded, unsweetened coconut, plus 2 teaspoons for topping

1. Combine all the ingredients in a blender. Pulse until creamy.
2. Divide the mixture among two pina colada glasses. Spread remaining 2 teaspoons of shredded coconut on top.
3. Serve immediately.

Chocolate Brownie Whoopie

1 Fueling | ½ Healthy Fat | 1 Condiment | 1 Optional Snack Prep
time: 10 minutes | Cook time: 18 minutes | Serves 2

2 sachets Optavia Decadent Double Chocolate Brownie

6 tablespoons unsweetened almond milk, divided

3 tablespoons liquid egg substitute

¼ teaspoon baking powder

1 teaspoon vegetable oil

¼ cup powdered peanut butter

Cooking spray

1. Preheat the oven to 350ºF (180ºC).

2. In a bowl, combine the Decadent Double Chocolate Brownie, ¼ cup almond milk, egg substitute, baking powder, and vegetable oil. Stir to mix well.

3. Divide the Chocolate Brownie batter among 4 slots of a greased muffin tin.

4. Bake in the preheated oven for 18 minutes or until a toothpick inserted in the center comes out clean.

5. Meanwhile, combine the powdered peanut butter and remaining almond milk in a small bowl.

6. When baking is complete, allow to cool, then slice each muffin in half horizontally.

7. Spread 1 tablespoon of peanut butter mixture on the bottom half of each muffin, then top with the remaining muffin halves.

8. Serve immediately.

Sweet Potato Muffins with Pecans

1 Fueling | 1 Healthy Fat | 1 Condiment

Prep time: 15 minutes | Cook time: 20 minutes | Serves 4

2 sachets Optavia Select Honey Sweet Potatoes

2 sachets OPTAVA Essential Spiced Gingerbread

¼ cup unsweetened almond milk

6 tablespoons liquid egg substitute

½ teaspoon pumpkin pie spice

½ teaspoon baking powder

½ teaspoon vanilla extract

1 cup water

1 ½ ounces (43 g) chopped pecans

Cooking Spray

1. Preheat the oven to 350ºF (180ºC).

2. Cook the Honey Sweet Potatoes according to the package directions. Allow to cool before using.

3. Combine the cooked Honey Sweet Potatoes with remaining ingredients, except for the pecans in a large bowl.

4. Divide the mixture among 8 slots of a greased muffin pan. Sprinkle with pecans on top.

5. Bake in the preheated oven for 20 minutes or until a toothpick inserted in the center comes out clean.

6. Serve immediately.

Blueberry Almond Flaxseed Scones

1 Fueling | 2 Healthy Fats | 2 Condiments

Prep time: 15 minutes | Cook time: 15 minutes | Serves 4

4 sachets Optavia Blueberry Almond Hot Cereal

¼ cup ground flaxseeds

2 packets stevia

½ teaspoon baking powder

3 tablespoons unsalted butter, frozen and cut into ½-inch pieces

3 tablespoons liquid egg white

3 tablespoons plain, low-fat Greek yogurt

¼ teaspoon cinnamon

1. Preheat the oven to 400ºF (205ºC).
2. Add the Blueberry Almond Hot Cereal, ground flaxseeds, stevia, and baking powder to a food processor. Pulse until smooth.
3. Add the frozen butter and pulse until mixture resembles a coarse meal.
4. Add the egg white and Greek yogurt, and pulse until the dough is sanity.
5. Form the dough into a 6-inch circle, then transfer the dough onto a parchment-lined baking sheet. Sprinkle with cinnamon.
6. Bake in the preheated oven for 15 minutes or until lightly browned.
7. After baking, allow to cool before cutting into eight wedges, then serve.

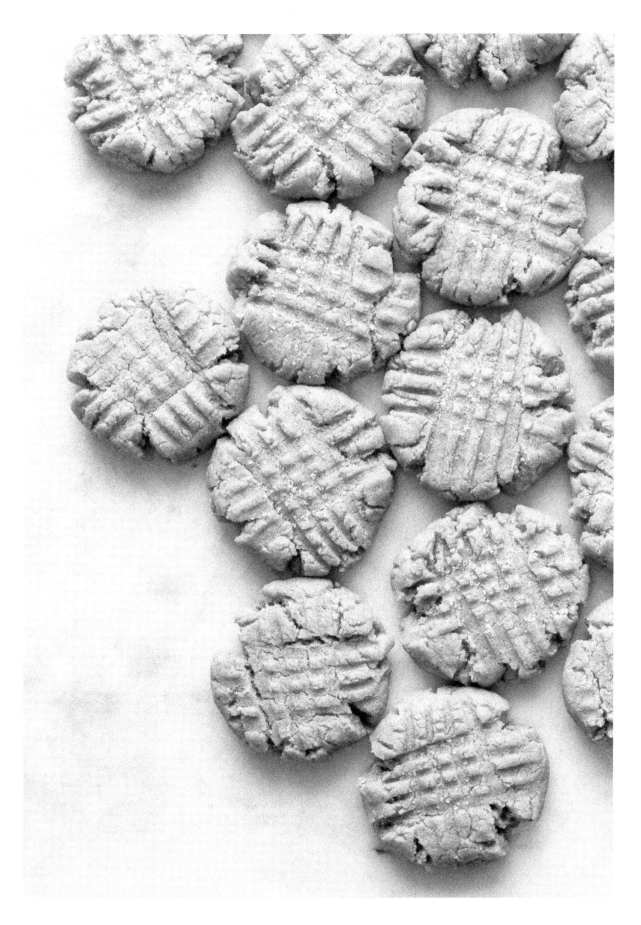

Peanut Butter Cookies

1 Fueling | ½ Healthy Fat | ½ Condiment

Prep time: 10 minutes | Cook time: 15 minutes | Serves 4

4 sachets Optavia Essential Silky Peanut Butter Shake

¼ cup unsweetened almond milk

1 tablespoon butter, melted

¼ teaspoon vanilla extract

¼ teaspoon baking powder

⅛ teaspoon sea salt

Cooking Spray

1. Preheat the oven to 350ºF (180ºC).

2. Combine all the ingredients, except the sea salt, in a large bowl and keep whisking until a sanity dough forms.

3. Scoop out dough into 8 balls with a cookie scoop. Arrange the balls on a foil-lined, greased baking sheet.

4. Flatten the mounds to create a criss-cross pattern with a fork. Sprinkle with salt.

5. Bake in the preheated oven for 15 minutes or until lightly browned.

6. Serve immediately.

Cinnamon French Toast Sticks

1 Fueling | 3 Condiments

Prep time: 5 minutes | Cook time: 8 minutes | Serves 2

2 sachets Optavia Essential Cinnamon Crunchy O's Cereal

2 tablespoons low-fat cream cheese, softened

6 tablespoons liquid egg substitute

Cooking spray

1. Put the Cinnamon Crunchy O's in a blender. Pulse until it has a breadcrumb-like consistency.

2. Pour in the cream cheese and liquid egg substitute, and pulse until a sanity dough forms.

3. Divide and shape the dough into 6 French toast stick pieces.

4. Spritz a skillet with cooking spray. Heat over medium high heat and cook the French toast sticks for 8 minutes on all sides or until lightly browned.

5. Serve immediately.

Hearty Zombie Frappe

1 Fueling | 3 Condiments

Prep time: 15 minutes | Cook time: 0 minutes | Serves 1

1 sachet Optavia Essential Creamy Vanilla Shake

1 cup unsweetened almond milk

1 tablespoon caramel syrup

½ cup ice

McCormick Color From Nature Food Colors- blue, yellow, and red

2 tablespoons plain, low-fat Greek yogurt

1 tablespoon unsweetened vanilla milk

2 tablespoons pressurized whipped topping

1. Put the Creamy Vanilla Shake, almond milk, caramel syrup, and ice in a blender. Pulse until smooth.

2. Add equal portions of blue and yellow food coloring until the shade of green is achieved.

3. In a bowl, mix the Greek yogurt and equal portions of blue and red food coloring until the shade of purple is achieved.

4. In a separate bowl, mix the vanilla milk with equal portions of blue and red food coloring until the shade of purple is achieved.

5. Drizzle purple Greek yogurt mixture down the sides of a cup. Fill cup with green shake mixture. Top with whipped topping and sprinkle with purple milk mixture.

6. Serve immediately.

Measurement Conversion Chart

VOLUME EQUIVALENTS(DRY)

US STANDARD	METRIC (APPROXIMATE)
1/8 teaspoon	0.5 mL
1/4 teaspoon	1 mL
1/2 teaspoon	2 mL
3/4 teaspoon	4 mL
1 teaspoon	5 mL
1 tablespoon	15 mL
1/4 cup	59 mL
1/2 cup	118 mL
3/4 cup	177 mL
1 cup	235 mL
2 cups	475 mL
3 cups	700 mL
4 cups	1 L

VOLUME EQUIVALENTS(LIQUID)

US STANDARD	US STANDARD (OUNCES)	METRIC (APPROXIMATE)
2 tablespoons	1 fl.oz.	30 mL
1/4 cup	2 fl.oz.	60 mL
1/2 cup	4 fl.oz.	120 mL
1 cup	8 fl.oz.	240 mL
1 1/2 cup	12 fl.oz.	355 mL
2 cups or 1 pint	16 fl.oz.	475 mL
4 cups or 1 quart	32 fl.oz.	1 L
1 gallon	128 fl.oz.	4 L

TEMPERATURES EQUIVALENTS

FAHRENHEIT(F)	CELSIUS(C) (APPROXIMATE)
225 °F	107 °C
250 °F	120 °C
275 °F	135 °C
300 °F	150 °C
325 °F	160 °C
350 °F	180 °C
375 °F	190 °C
400 °F	205 °C
425 °F	220 °C
450 °F	235 °C
475 °F	245 °C
500 °F	260 °C

WEIGHT EQUIVALENTS

US STANDARD	METRIC (APPROXIMATE)
1 ounce	28 g
2 ounces	57 g
5 ounces	142 g
10 ounces	284 g
15 ounces	425 g
16 ounces (1 pound)	455 g
1.5 pounds	680 g
2 pounds	907 g

CPSIA information can be obtained
at www.ICGtesting.com
Printed in the USA
BVHW011939050521
606335BV00017B/1013

Vampire Movies Quizzes & Trivia

Writen by:
David Crane, Marta Kauffman, Scott Silveri, Andrew
Reich, Alexa Junge, Jeff Greenstein, Jeff Strauss

MARIAN HAMADA

VAMPIRE

How well do you know your Vampire : Have you binge watched all
ten seasons? **Vampire & Trivia** is a fun Trivia for the TV series
fans. Test yourself of how much do you remember and how much
a fan of the Vampire TV series you are with this Vampire Trivia
Game. With questions and random difficulty levels, **Vampire
Quizzes & Trivia**, is the latest version of the trivia game card that
brings up and test your knowledge about the most loved TV
series. Take this game to prove whether or not you're a *true* fan.

QUIZ 1 - Vampire Movies Trivia

1. What vampire movie franchise features the character of Edward Cullen?
2. What vampire movie's tagline is "Forever.Begins.Now."?
3. "30 Days Of Night" is set in a small town in what often frozen state?
4. Who played the role of Dracula in "Dracula 2000"?
5. Who wants Lestat to be her king in "Queen of the Damned"?
6. What old and powerful vampire targets Buffy?
7. Who played Lothos in "Buffy, The Vampire Slayer"?
8. Who plays the role of Dracula in "The Satanic Rites of Dracula"?
9. What is monster-hunter Van Helsing's first name?
10. In the 2003 movie, "Underworld", what are the brutal Lycans?
11. Who starred in the lead role of Peter Loew in "Vampire's Kiss"?
12. What vampire movie opens with Count Dracula saying "Children of the night, shut up!"?
13. Who was cast as the child, Claudia, in "Interview With A Vampire"?
14. What blood-thirsty seductress was resurrected in "Bordello of Blood"?
15. In what movie does the Toronto vampire Boya fall in love with donut shop waitress, Molly?

Quiz 1 – Answers

1. Twilight

2. Twilight

3. Alaska

4. Gerard Butler

5. Queen Akasha

6. Lothos

7. Rutger Hauer

8. Christopher Lee

9. Gabriel

10. Werewolves

11. Nicolas Cage

12. Love At First Bite

13. Kirsten Dunst

14. Lilith

15. Blood & Donuts

QUIZ 2 - Vampire Movies Quiz

1. Who wrote the book upon which the 2002 movie "Queen of the Damned" is based?
2. Who is vampire hunter Nick after in "The Forsaken"?
3. What is the name of the town outcast who ultimately befriends Buffy?
4. Besides fighting vampires, what other extra-curricular activity is Buffy involved in?
5. Who played the role of Buffy in the 1992 movie "Buffy, The Vampire Slayer"?
6. What "Beverly Hills 90210" star played the role of Buffy's friend, Pike?
7. Who turned African prince Mamuwalde into "Blacula" in the 1972 movie?
8. Who played the title role in "Van Helsing"?
9. Who played the role of vampire warrior Selene in the movie "Underworld"?
10. Who starred as Count Dracula in the 1979 vampire-spoof "Love At First Bite"?
11. Who directed the 1995 film "Dracula: Dead and Loving It"?
12. Who played Blade, the half-vampire, half-mortal vampire slayer?
13. Who wrote the book upon which the 1979 movie "Salem's Lot" is based?
14. Who played the role of Louis de Pointe du Lac in the movie "Interview With A Vampire"?
15. What writer was initially unhappy with the casting of Tom Cruise as Lestat de Lioncourt?

Quiz 2 – Answers

1. Anne Rice

2. The Bloodletters

3. Pike

4. Cheerleading

5. Kristi Swanson

6. Luke Perry

7. Count Dracula

8. Hugh Jackman

9. Kate Beckinsale

10. George Hamilton

11. Mel Brooks

12. Wesley Snipes

13. Stephen King

14. Brad Pitt

15. Anne Rice

QUIZ 3 - Vampire Movies Trivia Questions & Answers : Horror Mixture

1. Who played the character who fought vampires in "The Last Man on Earth" (1964)?
2. What performer from "Last of the Summer Wine" played a man who got a stake through the heart in "Taste the Blood of Dracula"?
3. What director played a vampire hunter in "The Fearless Vampire Killers"?
4. In which of these movies was Dracula (Lon Chaney Jr) stranded after his coffin was burned?
5. What was the name of the vampire depicted in F. W. Murnau's 1922 film "Nosferatu: A Symphony of Horror"?
6. By almost any reckoning, the most influential vampire movie of all time was Universal Studios' "Dracula", from 1931. From innumerable remakes, to the Count character on "Sesame Street", this film cast the mold for how a vampire was supposed to look, sound, and act. Who played the title role in this groundbreaking work?
7. In 1931, the battle between Dracula and Van Helsing was brought to the big screen in Universal's "Dracula". Bela Lugosi was Count Dracula, but who played Dr. Van Helsing?
8. Rock star, 'Come out, come out... Wherever you are!?
9. Born in 1922 in London, England, Christopher Lee will always be remembered as the actor who 'revamped' the myth of Dracula. Very tall and handsome, he added to the character a touch of seduction greatly appreciated by the Count's fans. In which of these movies did he make his debut as the famous vampire?
10. What actor is the best-known for portraying Dracula?
11. Who played a character who collected blood for a monster in "The Vampire Bat"?

Quiz 3 – Answers

1. Vincent Price

2. Peter Sallis

3. Roman Polanski

4. Son of Dracula

5. Count Orlok

6. Bela Lugosi

7. Edward Van Sloan

8. Queen of the Damned

9. 'Dracula' or 'The Horror Of Dracula'

10. Bela Lugosi

11. Lionel Atwill

QUIZ 4 - At Dawn They Sleep

1. What was the name of the vampire depicted in F. W. Murnau's 1922 film "Nosferatu: A Symphony of Horror"?
2. Tod Browning's 1931 version of "Dracula" featured which famous actor in the titular role?
3. Remade by Hammer Horror in 1958, "Dracula" starred Christopher Lee in the title role. What was the alternate title for this shot-in-color film, which originally received an X-rating in the UK?
4. Directed by Mario Bava in 1960, what film originally made in Italian featured Barbara Steele in two roles - those of the main protagonist, Katia, and the vampiric antagonist, Asa Vadja?
5. The 1978 vampire film "Martin" was a significant independent addition to the genre directed by which filmmaker who was (perhaps) better-known for his zombie movies?
6. "The Lost Boys" (1987) featured teenage vampires and teenage vampire hunters in which otherwise normal locale?
7. In Kathryn Bigelow's "Near Dark" (1987), what happened to vampires who came into contact with sunlight?
8. The 1994 film "Interview With a Vampire" was originally based on a novel written by which famous horror author?
9. Quentin Tarantino and George Clooney were the Gecko Brothers in what 1996 film about a vampire strip club in Mexico?
10. Which one of these films from the 2000s/2010s did NOT involve vampires?

Quiz 4 – Answers

1. Count Orlok

2. Bela Lugosi

3. Horror of Dracula

4. Black Sunday

5. George A. Romero

6. California

7. They set ablaze

8. Anne Rice

9. From Dusk Till Dawn

10. Resident Evil

QUIZ 5 - Vampire Movies

1. What actor is the best-known for portraying Dracula?
2. In this 1987 movie, two brothers move to California, where they meet a group of young vampires. Starring Kiefer Sutherland and Jason Patric?
3. A vampire invades a small town in Maine in this movie based on a Stephen King novel?
4. Who played Dracula in 1992's 'Bram Stoker's Dracula'?
5. This 1992 British film, starring Julian Sands is loosely based on 'Annabel Lee' by Edgar Allan Poe?
6. This 1983 cult classic was based on a book by Whitley Streiber. It stars David Bowie and Susan Sarandon?
7. This 1922 silent German movie was banned for many years due to a lawsuit brought by Bram Stoker's widow.?
8. This 1994 movie, based on an Anne Rice novel stars Tom Cruise and Brad Pitt?
9. Not technically a 'vampire movie', it's about plant that drinks blood?
10. This 1970 movie starring Ingrid Pitt is probably the most faithful adaptation of 'Carmilla' by Sheridan Le Fanu?

Quiz 5 – Answers

1. Lugosi

2. Lost Boys

3. Salem's Lot

4. Gary Oldman

5. Tale of a Vampire

6. Hunger

7. Nosferatu, Eine Symphonie des Grauens

8. Interview with a Vampire

9. Little Shop of Horrors

10. The Vampire Lovers

QUIZ 6 - Vampires At The Movies

1. Born in 1922 in London, England, Christopher Lee will always be remembered as the actor who 'revamped' the myth of Dracula. Very tall and handsome, he added to the character a touch of seduction greatly appreciated by the Count's fans. In which of these movies did he make his debut as the famous vampire?

2. In most of the movies about Count Dracula, the character of R.M. Renfield occupies an important place because of his prophetic behavior announcing the coming of his Master, Dracula. Which of this actor never played Renfield?

3. Who played Professor Van Helsing in the 1979 version of 'Dracula' directed by John Badham?

4. In 'Interview With A Vampire', Claudia, the child vampire, is played by Kirsten Dunst. Which of these actresses auditioned for the role but, obvioulsy, did not get it?

5. In the poetic and absolutely beautiful 'The Wisdom Of Crocodile' (1998), Jude Law plays a modern vampire who feeds on the emotions of the woman he loves (before feeding more conservatively...). Which of these actresses did he save when she was about to throw herself in front of a train?

6. In John Carpenter's 'Vampires' (1998), Valek, the Master Vampire, is played by Thomas Ian Griffith. For how many years has Valek been a vampire?

7. In the very original 'Near Dark' (1987) directed by Kathryn Bigelow, by which of thse characters is the hero, Caleb (Adrian Pasdar), bitten?

Quiz 6 – Answers

1. 'Dracula' or 'The Horror Of Dracula'

2. Peter Fonda

3. Laurence Olivier

4. Christina Ricci

5. Kerry Fox

6. 600

7. Mae

QUIZ 8 – House of Vampires

1. What director played a vampire hunter in "The Fearless Vampire Killers"?
2. What performer from "...And Justice For All" played a vampire in "Saturday the 14th"?
3. What performer from "Enter the Dragon" met a vampire from another planet in "Queen of Blood"?
4. What performer from "Petticoat Junction" met a vampire in "Blood Bath"?
5. What performer from "Wildcats" fought vampires in "Blade"?
6. What performer from the movie "The Beverly Hillbillies" met vampires in "Bordello of Blood" (1996)?
7. What performer from "Child's Play" played a vampire in "Fright Night"?
8. What performer from "Cape Fear" fought vampires in "From Dusk Till Dawn"?
9. Who directed the vampire movie "Martin"?
10. Who played the lead vampire woman in "Vamp" (1986)?

Quiz 8 – Answers

1. Roman Polanski

2. Jeffrey Tambor

3. John Saxon

4. Lori (aka Linda) Saunders

5. Wesley Snipes

6. Erika Eleniak

7. Chris Sarandon

8. Juliette Lewis

9. George Romero

10. Grace Jones

QUIZ 9 – Dracula and Van Helsing in Films

1. In 1931, the battle between Dracula and Van Helsing was brought to the big screen in Universal's "Dracula". Bela Lugosi was Count Dracula, but who played Dr. Van Helsing?

2. Did Bela Lugosi, who played Count Dracula in Universal's 1931 horror hit "Dracula", appear in the studio's 1936 sequel called "Dracula's Daughter"?

3. Unfortunately, there was no Van Helsing to keep Dracula and his friends, the Wolf Man and the Frankenstein's Monster, from running amuck in "House of Frankenstein" (1944). Who played Count Dracula?

4. In what 1943 Lon Chaney Jr. movie did Count Alucard ('Dracula' spelled backwards) move from the Old World to seek romance and fresh blood in the American Deep South?

5. Who played Van Helsing in Hammer's 1958 film "Dracula" (aka "Horror of Dracula"), which starred Christopher Lee as Dracula?

6. T/F: Laurence Olivier played Prof. Abraham Van Helsing in "Dracula" (1979), which starred Frank Langella as Dracula.

7. After being evicted from Castle Dracula to make way for the Romanian gymnastic team, Count Dracula (George Hamilton) emigrated to New York City in pursuit of his true love, Cindy Sondheim (Susan Saint James), in what 1979 spoof?

Quiz 9 – Answers

1. Edward Van Sloan

2. N

3. John Carradine

4. Son of Dracula

5. Peter Cushing

6. T

7. Love At First Bite

QUIZ 10 – Ape About Dracula

1. In which of these movies was Dracula (Lon Chaney Jr) stranded after his coffin was burned?
2. In which of these movies did Dracula need virgin blood?
3. In which of these movies did Dracula kill someone and then seduce the man's granddaughter-in-law?
4. In the movie "Blood of Dracula's Castle" who played as Dracula's butler?
5. In which movie was Dracula impaled on a cross?
6. In which of these movies was Dracula resurrected after someone drank Dracula's blood?
7. In which of these movies was Dracula struck by lightning?
8. In which of these movies did Dracula fall on stakes?
9. In which movie did Lionel Atwill play as Inspector Holtz?
10. In the movie "Dracula: Dead and Loving It", who played as Dr. Van Helsing?
11. Which of the following countries does not border Count Dracula's castle?
12. Who warns Jonathan Harker, as he approaches Castle Dracula, "Do you not know that tonight, when the clock strikes midnight, all the evil things in the world will have full sway"?
13. Which of the following descriptions is not applied to Dracula?
14. What is the name of the ship on which Dracula travels to England, which is found empty of crew, with just one body remaining?
15. What does Renfield, the insane man with a strange connection to Dracula, eat?

Quiz 10 – Answers

1. Son of Dracula

2. Andy Warhol's Dracula

3. House of Frankenstein

4. John Carradine

5. Dracula Has Risen From the Grave (1968)

6. Taste the Blood of Dracula

7. Scars of Dracula

8. Dracula A.D. 1972

9. House of Dracula

10. Mel Brooks

11. Hungary

12. The landlady at his hotel

13. Blood-red eyes

14. The Demeter

15. Spiders, flies and sparrows

QUIZ 11 - Ape About Dracula II

1. What performer from "Last of the Summer Wine" played a man who got a stake through the heart in "Taste the Blood of Dracula"?
2. Who played Dracula in "Love At First Bite"?
3. Who played Prince Mamuwalde in "Blacula" (1972)?
4. Which Dracula movie had a couple named Charles and Diana?
5. In which movie did Dracula lose his arms and legs, but he was still alive?
6. Who played Dracula in "Count Dracula's Great Love" (1974)?
7. What performer from "Superman Returns" played as Dracula in "Dracula" (1979)?
8. Who played Dracula in "Brides of Dracula"?
9. Who played Van Helsing's granddaughter in "Dracula A.D. 1972"?
10. Who played Van Helsing's granddaughter in "The Satanic Rites of Dracula"?
11. Who is Dracula said to have been inspired by?
12. In what disguise does Dracula first meet Harker?
13. Who is the "bloofer lady" who preys on small children?
14. From where does Abraham van Helsing arrive to help fight the plague of vampires?
15. How is Dracula finally killed?

Quiz 11 – Answers

1. Peter Sallis

2. George Hamilton

3. William Marshall

4. Dracula: Prince of Darkness

5. Andy Warhol's Dracula

6. Paul Naschy

7. Frank Langella

8. Nobody

9. Stephanie Beacham

10. Joanna Lumley

11. Henry Irving, Bram Stoker's boss at London's Lyceum Theatre

12. A coachman

13. Lucy

14. Amsterdam

15. He is slashed through the throat with one knife and simultaneously stabbed in the heart with another

QUIZ 12 - World of Vampires

1. Who played the character who fought vampires in "The Last Man on Earth" (1964)?
2. Who played a character who collected blood for a monster in "The Vampire Bat"?
3. Who played the title role in "Vampire in Brooklyn"?
4. Who played the character who fought vampires in "The Omega Man" (1971)?
5. Who played the character who fought vampires in "I Am Legend" (2007)?
6. Who played the vampire who became old waiting to see the doctor in "The Hunger" (1983)?
7. Who played a character who created a vampire in "Scream and Scream Again"?
8. Who played Dracula in "Blood of Dracula's Castle"?
9. Who burned Dracula in "Dracula's Daughter" (1936)?
10. Who played Dr. Van Helsing in "House of Dracula"?
11. In Interview with the Vampire, who's the interviewee?
12. Who plays the leader of the vampires in Near Dark?
13. What's the title of George A. Romero's 1976 film about a teenager who believes he's a vampire?
14. Which of these isn't a real film?
15. Who was the original Buffy the Vampire Slayer?

Quiz 12 - Answers

1. Vincent Price

2. Lionel Atwill

3. Eddie Murphy

4. Charlton Heston

5. Will Smith

6. David Bowie

7. Vincent Price

8. Alex D'Arcy

9. Countess Zaleska

10. Nobody

11. Louis de Pointe du Lac (Brad Pitt)

12. Lance Henriksen

13. Martin

14. Dracula in Space

15. Kristy Swanson

QUIZ 13 - Vampire Trivia Quiz

1. Which of the following historical characters was the basis for some of today's vampire stories?
2. Published in 1887, which of the following authors penned the book "Dracula"?
3. What was the name of the vampire character that Brad Pitt played in the film "Interview with a Vampire - The Vampire Chronicles"?
4. Which spice is reputed to repel vampires?
5. What is a group of vampires called?
6. On which well-known television series might you see Count von Count?
7. Dating from the early Neolithic period (4000 to 3000 BC), what is a dolmen?
8. What animal can Chinese vampires transform into?
9. Found in popular Chinese mythology, what does Chiang Shih translate to?
10. What was the first film to feature vampires?
11. What was the name of the female vampire in Joseph Sheridan Le Fanu's novel of the same name?
12. An unborn baby whose father is vampire is called what?
13. Which of these events might change a person into a vampire?
14. What kind of fruit did some people in the Balkans believe would turn into a vampire if not eaten before Christmas?
15. With many stories, which attribute to her vampire-like tendencies, where did Elizabeth Bathory call home?

Quiz 13 – Answers

1. Vlad the Impaler

2. Bram Stoker

3. Louis

4. Garlic

5. A clutch

6. Sesame Street

7. A stone monument

8. Wolf

9. Corpse hopper

10. Secrets of House No. 5

11. Carmilla

12. Glogalve

13. A cat jumping on the body before burial

14. Watermelon

15. Hungary

QUIZ 14 - Vampires Quiz 1

1. Who is the creator of the character Count Dracula?
2. Dracula comes from the area called Transylvania. In which country is transylvania?
3. Who is the arch rival of Count Dracula?
4. On who is the character Dracula allegedly based?
5. On his death which famous horror film star was buried in his Dracula costume?
6. Which famous british actor portrayed dracula in the video to pet shop boys song Heart?
7. What film is generally regarded as the very first vampire movie?
8. Which British film company was responsible for the production of many of the vampire movies of the 60?s and 70?s?
9. Which actor does the interviewing in the film Interview with a Vampire?
10. What is the name of Dracula?s insane henchman? Is it Vladimir, Renfield, Victor, Karlof or Bill?
11. Vampire comes from the Albanian word 'dhampir', which means what?
12. How do people turn into vampires?
13. In which year did the word 'vampire' appear in the Oxford Dictionary?

Quiz 14 – Answers

1. Bram Stoker

2. Romania

3. Professor Von Helsing

4. Vlad the impaler

5. Bela Lugosi

6. Ian McKellen

7. Nosferatu (1921)

8. Hammer Films

9. Christian Slater

10. Renfield

11. To drink with teeth

12. After being bitten by one

13. 1734

QUIZ 15 - How Well Do You Know "The Lost Boys"

1. How do the Frog brothers learn about vampires?
2. What happens when Michael follows the gang on a motorcycle?
3. How does Sam realize Michael is turning into a vampire?
4. When Michael and Sam hang out on the boardwalk, they see _____ posters.?
5. What does the gang fill their water guns with?
6. Who else is a half-vampire?
7. The Chinese food the motorcycle gang gets turns into _____.?
8. What does the gang have to do to turn Michael back into a human?
9. Who turns out to be the head vampire?
10. How does the head vampire die?
11. Where did the Frog brothers move from?
12. Why was Max dating Lucy?
13. Who was supposed to be Star's first kill?
14. How many half-vampires are there?
15. What must a half-vampire do to become a full vampire?

Quiz 15 – Answers

1. Comic Books

2. He almost goes over a cliff

3. His reflection in the mirror is transparent

4. Missing Person

5. Holy water

6. Star

7. Blood and Guts

8. Kill the "head" vampire

9. Max

10. Grandpa crashes his jeep into him

11. Arizona

12. He wanted a mother for his "lost boys"

13. Michael

14. Three

15. Kill someone

QUIZ 17 - the-vampire-diaries

1. 'The Vampire Diaries' is actually based on a book by the same name. What is the name of the author?
2. When did 'The Vampire Diaries' first air?
3. In the pilot of 'The Vampire Diaries', we're introduced to the talented cast. What is the name of the actress that plays Vicki Donovan?
4. The pilot marks the seemingly endless love affair between Elena and Damon (Delena) when they meet for the first time.?
5. Mystic Falls is the main location for 'The Vampire Diaries' and the Gilberts are one of the founding families. How many founding families are there in total?
6. In which state is Mystic Falls located?
7. There are many deaths during 'The Vampire Diaries'. Jeremy is one of the main characters who ends up losing his life more than most. How many times does Jeremy die in those eight seasons?
8. Throughout 'The Vampire Diaries', there is an herb which allows humans to be protected from compulsion. What is it called?
9. Tyler Lockwood transitions into a werewolf due to his family curse. Why does Tyler reveal his true self to his mother?
10. Stefan Salvatore is a heartthrob in Mystic Falls (and for fans). He also happens to have a few doppelgängers. How many?

Quiz 17 – Answers

1. L.J. Smith

2. September 10th, 2009

3. Kayla Ewell

4. False

5. 5

6. Virginia

7. 5

8. Vervain

9. To protect Caroline

10. 3

QUIZ 18 - Try Matching 100% Of These Characters To Their Vampire Movies And TV Shows

1. What Vampire Movie Stars Bella Swan?
2. What Vampire Show Is Stefan Salvatore From?
3. What Vampire Series Is Pamela Swynford De Beaufort From?
4. What Vampire Film Stars Edward Cullen?
5. What Show Features Buffy Summers?
6. What Show Features Elijah Mikaelson?
7. What Show Featured Bill Compton?
8. What Vampire Film Features Selene?
9. What Vampire Show Features Rebekah Mikaelson?
10. What Vampire Show Is Sookie Stackhouse From?
11. What Vampire Show Features Katherine Pierce?
12. What Vampire Film Features This Character?
13. What Vampire Show Is Eric Northman On?
14. What Vampire Film Features Lestat?
15. What Vampire Show Is Davina Claire From?

Quiz 18 – Answers

1. Twilight

2. The Vampire Diaries

3. True blood

4. The Twilight Saga

5. Buffy the Vampire Slayer

6. The Originals

7. True Blood

8. The Underworld Series

9. The Originals

10. True Blood

11. The Vampire Diaries

12. Blade

13. True Blood

14. Interview with a Vampire

15. The Originals

THE ONE WITH ALL THE QUESTIONS

QUIZ 19 - The Vampires

1. The legends of vampires originated in Africa.?
2. The belief in vampires resulted in a mass hysteria.?
3. Belief in vampires was an attempt of people of pre-industrial societies to explain the process of death and decomposition.?
4. What is the most common way of becoming a vampire?
5. Why don't vampires have a reflection and, in some cultures, don't even cast shadows?
6. John Polidori authored the first vampire story called:?
7. Bram Stoker's classic novel of horror "Dracula" introduced the vampire Count Dracula of:?
8. What is the correct name for this vampire-hunter TV show?
9. Which of these actors did not star in the 1994 movie "Interview with the Vampire"?
10. 'Vampire lifestyle' is a term for:?

Quiz 19 – Answers

1. False.

2. True.

3. True.

4. Being bitten by a vampire.

5. Because they lack a soul..

6. The Vampyre.

7. Transylvania.

8. Buffy the Vampire Slayer.

9. George Clooney.

10. A contemporary subculture of people.

QUIZ 20 - The Vampire Diaries Quiz

1. Why does Stefan seem to be interested in Elena in season 1?
2. Did Elena first meet Stefan or Damon?
3. At the ending of the 5th season, who does end up in the prison world?
4. How does Liv die at the ending of the 6th season?
5. How does Enzo die in the 8th season?
6. Which were the Founding Families of Mystic Falls?
7. Why did Johnathan Gilbert's devices actually work?
8. Why does Elena turn off her humanity in season 4?
9. What graduation gift does Klaus offer to Caroline?
10. Who carried Stefan's child?
11. Why was Caroline desperate to get Stefan's attention in the first episodes?
12. Why did Stefan turn off his humanity soon after Caroline turned hers?
13. What job did Stefan want to have before turning into a vampire?

Quiz 20 – Answers

1. She looked just like Katherine.

2. Damon.

3. Damon and Bonnie.

4. Tyler suffocates her.

5. Stefan rips his heart out.

6. Fell, Gilbert, Salvatore, Lockwood and Forbes.

7. Emily Bennet put her spell on them.

8. Jeremy dies

9. Tyler's freedom.

10. Valerie.

11. She felt like it was always Elena, but never her.

12. She would have killed his niece if he hadn't turned it off.

13. Doctor.

QUIZ 21 - The Ultimate Vampire Diaries Quiz

1. What state is Mystic Falls in?
2. In Season 1, how does Vicki die?
3. In Season 1, what really brings Alaric to Mystic Falls?
4. What does the herb vervain do?
5. Why does Katherine turn Caroline into a vampire?
6. What's the purpose of the Gilbert ring?
7. In Season 2, why does Caroline end her relationship with Matt?
8. Who are The Originals?
9. What does the "Lockwood curse" say?
10. What happens when Katherine is injured?
11. In Season 2, why does Stefan join Klaus?
12. In Season 3, how does Matt connect to Vicki's ghost?
13. Why does Tyler finally tell his mother he's a werewolf?
14. What powers does Elena's necklace have?
15. In Season 2, why is Klaus tracking Elena?

Quiz 21 – Answers

1. Virginia

2. Stefan is forced to stake her

3. He wants to avenge his wife's death.

4. It protects humans from vampire compulsion

5. So she can sacrifice her to Klaus.

6. It protects the wearer from death by supernatural causes

7. She fed off him and feels guilty

8. The first generation of vampires

9. In order to become a werewolf, Tyler must kill somebody.

10. Elena is also injured

11. To save Elena

12. Through Jeremy's new powers

13. To convince her to free Caroline

14. It can contact the Original Witch.

15. He wants to use her blood to create more hybrids.

QUIZ 22 - Vampire-Diaries-Trivia-Quiz

1. In what town does the show primarily take place?
2. How many seasons was the show on TV?
3. What is the name Stefan's best friend, who appears in season one and is promptly killed?
4. Tyler is a hybrid — a vampire and what?
5. What is Katherine's real name?
6. In what season does Elena become a vampire?
7. What is the herb called that can protect you from being compelled by a vampire?
8. Who is Stefan's evil doppelgänger?
9. When Damon and Bonnie are trapped in the prison world with Kai Parker, the same day keeps repeating over and over. What is the date?
10. How does Liz Forbes die?
11. Who saves Elena from the car accident that killed her parents?
12. What does Bonnie call her grandmother?
13. What are the names of Alaric's twin daughters?
14. What is the Staff of Arcadius?
15. What is the last name of the original vampire family?

Quiz 22 – Answers

1. Mystic Falls

2. 8

3. Lexi

4. Werewolf

5. Katerina

6. 4

7. Vervain

8. Silas

9. May 10, 1994

10. Cancer

11. Stefan

12. Grams

13. Lizzie and Josie

14. Tuning fork

15. Mikaelson

QUIZ 23 - vampires-101

1. in what year did stefan and damon become vampires?
2. which of the salvatore brothers first became a vampire?
3. Which of these characters did we first see turn into a vampire?
4. Damon tries to get Elena to kiss him but is stopped by what?
5. who helps Bonnie learn magic and helps her open and close the tomb?
6. in which season do we see elena turn her humanity off?
7. which character is Silas's doppelganger?
8. true or false? in a season we learn that Vicki is still alive?
9. which of these are Elena's BIRTH parents?
10. which of these characters is NOT an original?
11. which girl was crowned miss mystic falls?
12. what is the name of the continuous dance every year?

Quiz 23 – Answers

1. 1864

2. stefan

3. Caroline

4. Vervain in her necklace

5. her grandmother

6. 4th

7. stefan

8. False

9. isobel and john

10. Kathrine

11. caroline

12. decade dance

QUIZ 24 - The Great Vampire Films

1. By almost any reckoning, the most influential vampire movie of all time was Universal Studios' "Dracula", from 1931. From innumerable remakes, to the Count character on "Sesame Street", this film cast the mold for how a vampire was supposed to look, sound, and act. Who played the title role in this groundbreaking work?

2. Sexuality and passion have always been prominent in the vampire mythos, and this 1983 film starring Catherine Deneuve and Susan Sarandon is no exception. Based on a novel by Whitley Streiber, what is the name of this movie that continues to raise eyebrows?

3. When making "Dracula" in 1931, Universal Studios experimented with an alternative to foreign language dubbing: when the English-speaking cast went home for the night, a Spanish-speaking cast would take over, filming their own movie on the very same sets. The two films are similar, but the Spanish version (directed by George Melford) differs from the English in many ways. Which of these is NOT a substantial difference between the two versions?

4. Starring cult-film mainstay Barbara Steele as a Russian witch who is executed in 1630 - only to return for bloody vengence 200 years later - this 1960 picture was banned in the UK for eight years due to its graphic imagery and subject matter. What was this controversial amalgamation of fantastic imagery directed by Italian legend Mario Bava?

Quiz 24 – Answers

1. Bela Lugosi

2. The Hunger

3. In the Spanish version, star Carlos Villarias is outfitted with a fine set of fangs, unlike his English-version counterpart who goes au naturelle.

4. Black Sunday

QUIZ 25 - Vampire Academy Quiz

1. What is Dimitri surname?

2. Where is St. Vladimir's Academy located?

3. Who is the male friend of Rose's who has a crush on her?

4. In Frostbite, which royal Moroi whom Rose met and seemed to be stalking her?

5. Which female seemed to have a more-than-friends relationship with Dimitri in Frostbite?

6. Which royal Moroi family was Rose's mother, Janine Hathaway, guarding?

7. In Shadow Kiss, it is known that Adrian is a relation of the queen. What is his relation to her?

8. The Queen has a secret dhampir lover. What is his name?

9. Whose ghost guided Rose and told her of the Strigoi whereabouts and later, Dimitri's fate?

10. And finally, the most painful question of all. What happened to Dimitri at the end of Shadow Kiss?

Quiz 25 – Answers

1. Belikov

2. Montana

3. Mason Ashford

4. Adrian Ivashkov

5. Tasha Ozera

6. Szelsky

7. Great nephew

8. Ambrose

9. Mason Ashford

10. Was turned into a Strigoi

The One With All the Cards – Vampire – Box Against Vampire

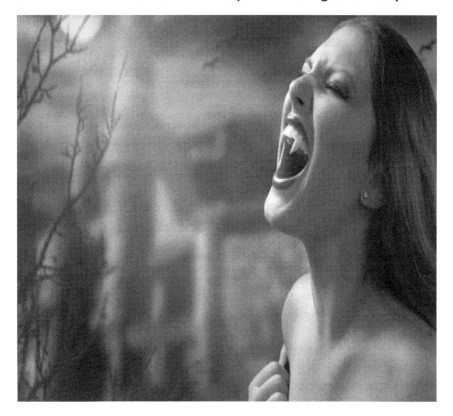

https://boxgamefun.com/

Printed in Great Britain
by Amazon

24447369R00029